The
SIRTFOOD
Diet

For those who want to lose weight quickly and burn fat without giving up some of their favorite foods, with the revolutionary diet most loved by VIPs. Includes meal plan and recipes.

- Adele Goggins —

Legal Notice

Disclaimer Notice

TABLE OF CONTENTS

The Sirt Food diet: *For those who want to lose weight quickly and burn fat without giving up some of their favorite foods, with the revolutionary diet most loved by VIPs. Includes meal plan and recipes.*

Chapter 1: INTRODUCTION TO SIRTFOOD

What is Sirt Food?

Sirtfoods are recently found a group of nutrient-rich foods which appear to be able to actuate the body's skinny genes (otherwise called sirtuins), similarly as fasting diets do, with a similar scope of advantages, however without the regular drawbacks of fasting diets, for example, irritability, hunger, and muscle loss. By eating a diet rich in Sirtfoods, it is asserted that participants will get thinner, gain muscle, look, and feel good and possibly live a longer and increasingly healthy life.

What Is Sirt Food Diet?

The Sirtfood Diet is the better approach to move weight rapidly without radical dieting by initiating the same 'skinny gene' pathways generally just induced by fasting and exercise. Certain foods contain synthetic compounds called polyphenols that put mild stress on our phones, turning on genes that copy the impacts of exercise and fasting. Foods rich in polyphenols- including dark chocolate, kale, and red wine trigger the sirtuin pathways that affect digestion, mood, and aging. A diet rich in these sirtfoods launches weight reduction without sacrificing muscle while maintaining excellent health.

Add healthy sirtfoods to your diet for successful and sustained weight reduction, incredible vitality, and sparkling health. Switch on your body's fat-burning powers, supercharge weight reduction and help stave off disease with this simple-to-follow diet created by the specialists in nutritional prescription who proved the effect of Sirt foods. Dark chocolate, kale, coffee - these are foods that actuate sirtuins and switch on the alleged 'skinny gene' pathways in the body. The Sirtfood Diet gives you a straightforward, healthy way for eating for weight reduction, delicious simple-to-make plans, and a maintained plan for delayed success. The Sirtfood Diet is a diet of incorporation, not avoidance, and sirtfoods are widely affordable and available. This is a diet that urges you to get your fork and knife and appreciate eating delicious healthy food while seeing the wellbeing and weight reduction benefits.

The Origin Of Sirt food Diet

A couple of health experts called Glen Matten and Aidan Goggins, whose spotlight has consistently been on smart dieting as opposed to weight reduction. In their new book The Sirtfood Diet, the pair spread out a feast plan which includes drinking three sirtfood green squeezes a day joined by adjusted sirtfood-rich meals, for example, a buckwheat and prawn stir-fry or smoked salmon sirt super salad.

Power of Sirt Food

The Sirtfood Diet's authors make bold claims, including that the diet will induce supercharge weight loss, turn the "skinny gene" on and prevent disease. The thing is they don't have any evidence to back them up. There is no convincing evidence to date that the Sirtfood Diet has a more beneficial effect on weight loss than any other diet limited by calories.

Also, albeit huge numbers of those nourishments have healthy properties, no drawn-out human examinations have been conducted to decide if eating a diet rich in sirt nourishments has any substantial health advantages. However, a pilot study completed by the writers and involving 39 members from their fitness center is accounted for in the Sirtfood Diet book. Be that as it may, the aftereffects of this study doesn't appear to have been published elsewhere.

Participants followed the diet for a week and were walking every day. At the end of the week, participants lost a total of 7 pounds (3.2 kg) and retained or even added muscle mass. Those findings, however, are hardly shocking. Limiting your calorie intake to 1,000 calories, and actively exercising, would almost always induce weight loss. Regardless, this form of rapid weight loss is neither permanent nor long-lasting, and this research did not monitor participants beyond the first week to see whether they gained any of the weight back, as is normally the case.

As well as consuming fat and muscle, when the body is drained of energy, it uses its emergency energy reserves or glycogen. Every glycogen molecule requires 3–4 water molecules for storage. If your body uses glycogen, the water always gets rid of it. It is known as "weight in water." Only about one-third of the weight loss comes from fat during the first week of extreme calorie restriction, while the other two-thirds come from water, muscle, and glycogen. As soon as your calorie intake increases, your body replenishes its glycogen stores, and the weight comes right back. Unfortunately, this type of calorie restriction can also cause your body to lower its metabolic rate, causing you to need even fewer calories per day for energy than before. This diet may likely help you lose a few pounds in the beginning, but it will likely come back as soon as the diet is over.

As well as consuming fat and muscle, when the body is drained of energy, it uses its emergency energy reserves or glycogen. Each glycogen molecule requires 3–4 water molecules for storage. If your body uses glycogen, the water always gets rid of it. It is known as "weight in water." Pretty much 33% of the weight reduction originates from fat during the first week of extreme calorie limitation while the other 66% originate from skin, glycogen, and muscle. Your body will replenish its glycogen stores as soon as your calorie intake increases, and the weight returns right back. Unfortunately, this sort of calorie limitation can likewise make your body bring down its metabolic rate, causing energy requirements to be even lower in calories per day. This diet is likely to help you lose a few pounds in the beginning, but it'll probably return as soon as the diet is done.

As far as disease prevention is concerned, it is likely three weeks not long enough to have any meaningful long-term effects. On the other hand, it might very well be a smart idea to add sirtfood to your daily diet over the long term. But you might as well miss the diet in that scenario, and start doing it now. This eating regimen can assist you with getting thinner since it is low in calories, however when the diet finishes, the weight is probably going to return. The diet is too short even to consider impacting on your health over the long haul.

How it is better than other diet

Sirtfoods are a recently found group of regular plant foods, known as sirtuin activators, which switch on our 'skinny' qualities – similar qualities enacted by fasting and exercise. Unlike other diet plans, which are explicitly outfitted towards unhealthy and dramatic weight loss, the Sirtfood Diet is great if you essentially need to boost your resistant system, pack in certain nutrients, and feel somewhat healthier.

Alongside this fat-burning impact, sirtfoods additionally have the unique capacity to ¬naturally control hunger and increase muscle function – making them the ideal answer for accomplishing a healthy weight. Undoubtedly, their health-boosting impacts are incredible to such an extent that a few studies have shown them to be more powerful than professionally prescribed medications in forestalling constant infection, with apparent ¬benefits in diabetes, coronary illness, and ¬Alzheimer's disease. No big surprise cultures eating the most sirtfoods – including Italy and Japan – are the least fatty and most healthy on the planet. What's more, that is the reason we've formulated a diet based around them.

How Sirt Food diet works

The diet has two simple-to-follow phases:

PHASE 1 - This goes on for seven days. During the initial three days, you ought to have three sirtfood green juices and one full feast rich in sirtfoods – an aggregate of 1,000 calories. On days four to seven, you should expand your calorie admission to 1,500 by having two green juices and two meals day by day.

PHASE 2 - This 14-day maintenance phase is expected to assist you with getting more fit relentlessly. You can eat three balanced sirtfood-rich suppers consistently, in addition to one green juice. The two phases can be rehashed at whatever point you like for a fat-loss boost.

What occurs after the second phase? What's more, is this sort of diet extremely sustainable?

The idea of "sirtifying" dinners is for the individuals who have finished phase one and two yet at the same

15

time need to proceed on the Sirtfood path. It includes taking your preferred dish and giving it a Sirtfood contort. Recipes incorporate regular top picks, for example, chicken curry, bean stew con-Carne, pancakes, and pizza. The Sirtfood Diet isn't intended to be a one-off 'diet' yet rather a lifestyle. You are energized, when you've finished the initial three weeks, to continue on a diet rich in Sirtfoods and to continue drinking your daily green juice. There are presently various Sirtfood Diet recipe books accessible, with recipes for parcels more Sirtfood-rich primary dinners, just as recipes for options in contrast to the green juice and more tips and hints for following the Sirtfood Diet. There are even a couple of plans for Sirtfood treats! Phases one and two can be repeated as and when essential for a wellbeing boost, or if things have gone somewhat off course.

Who Sirt Food diet is for?

This diet seems to appear to spring up normally, and the Sirtfood Diet is one of the most recent which is for anyone and everyone that intends to drive their weight loss from fat and not muscle, ensure you look better, feel better and have more energy, prepare your body for long-term weight loss success. This eating regimen has gotten the biggest names in Europe and is well known for permitting chocolate and red wine.

The authors of the Sirtfood Diet make bold claims, including that the diet will induce supercharge weight loss, turn on the "skinny gene" and prevent illness. At the end of the week, participants lost an average of 7 pounds (3.2 kg) and maintained, or even gained, muscle mass. This diet may help you lose weight because it's low in calories, but the weight is likely to return when the diet ends. The diet is too short to have any long-term effect on your health.

Chapter 2:
SIRTUNIS AND SIRT DIETS

A diet highlighting dark chocolate, red wine, kale, berries, and coffee? Either it sounds like the best possible way to get well and lose weight, or it sounds too good to be true. However, it shows signs of improvement: These and other alleged "sirtfoods" should initiate the components constrained by the natural "skinny qualities" of your body to assist you with losing weight and burning fat, as per the makers of the Sirtfood Diet. What makes the Sirtfood Diet so powerful is their ability to switch to an ancient gene family that exists within each of us. The name for that gene family is sirtuin. Sirtuins are special because they orchestrate processes that affect important things like our ability to burn fat, our susceptibility — or not — to sickness, and eventually also to our futures. The effect of sirtuins is so profound that they are now referred to as "master metabolic regulators."

In essence, what exactly anyone who wants to shed some pounds and live a long and healthy life would want to be in charge of.

In recent years, sirtuins have, understandably, become the subject of intense scientific research. The first sirtuin was discovered in yeast back in 1984, and interest really began over the next three decades when it was revealed that sirtuin activation improves life span, first in yeast, and then all the way up to mice. Why the thrills? Since the fundamental concepts of cellular metabolism are almost similar from yeast to humans, and all in between. If you can manipulate anything as tiny as budding yeast and see a benefit, then replicate it in higher organisms like mice, there is potential for the same benefits to be realized in humans.

The Sirtfood Diet sounds obviously appealing, comprising a list of delightful foods you certainly already love and supported by claims that after having a daughter, Adele used it to lose weight. But here not to ruin your high chocolate-and-red-wine, but the evidence simply does not support the diet 's biggest claims. That is not to say eating sirt food is a bad idea. But as with all the diets that sound too good to be true, you should look at this one closely. Here's what you need to know about what sirtfoods can and can't do to you.

Behind the arguments of the benefits of sirtfoods, there is certain research, but it is very vague and rather contentious. Research at the sirt frontier is still super new. Studies investigate the role of the SIRT1 gene in aging and longevity, in weight gain associated with aging and age-related disease, and in protecting the heart against inflammation caused by a high-fat diet. But the study is limited to work done in test tubes and on mice, which is not sufficient evidence to suggest that sirtuin-boosting foods may have weight loss or anti-aging capabilities in a living, breathing human body.

Brooke Alpert, R.D., author of The Sugar Detox, says work indicates that sirtfood's weight-control benefits that come in part from the polyphenol-antioxidant resveratrol, which is sometimes hyped as an ingredient in red wine. "That said, it would be difficult to get benefits from drinking enough red wine," she says, adding that she also recommends resveratrol supplements to her customers.

Chapter 3
HOW TO FIGHT AGAINST OBESITY

Focus on the nutritional content of your food

Lack of a nutritious diet can cause obesity. You can reduce your calorie intake by making healthier choices and eating a balanced diet, and reduce the threat of obesity. Make sure you have plenty of fruits and vegetables in your shopping cart, so you can conveniently catch a piece of fruit or vegetable if hunger hits. You will target having five different pieces of fruit and vegetables every day.

Scan the food and beverage labels and find out exactly what's in them, so you can make educated choices when you purchase them. Be mindful of the calories you consume. You don't have to be on a diet, but knowing how many calories you eat will help you eat no more than your body needs. Eat smaller meals daily to avoid hunger because this helps keep your metabolism up without snacking foods with high sugar content. Don't feel the urge to finish everything on your plate if you start feeling full. Swap junk foods, processed foods, and takeaways for healthier substitutes. Don't store at home unhealthy choices. Make healthier choices when eating out. Numerous cafés now detail their meals' calories and dietary substances, and that will assist you with settling on an informed choice.

Avoid unhealthy and sugar-laden drinks

Numerous delicate and alcoholic drinks have high sugar content. An excess of sugar can prompt weight gain and obesity. In split second powdered beverages, squashes, juice drinks, and fizzy drinks that contain a great deal of added sugar, however, not many supplements. Natural fruit juices and smoothies are frequently thought to be a solid option, but they contain sugar, so you ought to confine your admission to a joined aggregate of 150ml per day. You will strive to drink about 6 to 8 glasses of fluid a day. Water is best, and it's a healthy, inexpensive choice to quench your thirst. It does not have any calories, but sugars. Other healthier options include lower fat milk and sugar-free beverages, including coffee and tea.

Alcohol calories are 'vacuum calories,' they have no nutritional value. Your body can't store alcohol, so processes like nutrient absorption and burning fat are interrupted to get rid of the alcohol. You can still drink alcohol, but you are aiming for less drink. Many alcoholic brands now have 'light' or low alcohol alternatives that can be tried or chosen for a low-calorie mixer like diet coke. Drinking water in alcoholic drinks will cut down on the number of units you consume.

Learn about and understand your eating habits

Research on obesity has found that obese people can suffer from many emotional problems regarding their weight and body image. Conversing with an expert about your eating pattern can regularly assist you with understanding them more, and with this information, you can find a way to beat gorging or eating solace. You can need to converse with a family member or friend and get from them the assist you with expecting to make them feel better.

Obesity treatment

If you are obese and have attempted to lose weight by diet and exercise, but have not reached or sustained a successful weight loss level, or you have a severe health problem that might be changed if you lose weight, such as type 2 diabetes or high blood pressure, then weight loss treatment or surgery may be the best choice for you.

How to beat obesity

Williamsburg, Va. — Experts agree: obesity in our nation has become an almost epidemic crisis. So at a ground-breaking obesity conference earlier this month, academic, health care, business, media, and policy leaders gathered to discuss solutions to the issue. The concept behind the Time / ABC News Conference on Obesity was to look from both angles at the problems. The aim was to encourage the participants to return and make a difference in their communities. So, what's the latest tactic in the obesity war? Here are a few accentuations:

Taking a Village — NOW!

In every talk, "Time is of the essence" was a message repeated as was the call for prevention — beginning with our children. Experts accepted that our children would be the original to die sooner than their parents due to the adult-like diseases that go along with obesity in their childhood. There's always been a consensus that working together is the best way to win the fight on obesity. If we are going to make a difference, the food industry, government, health care providers, students, neighborhoods, and parents all need to join hands. If we don't, we'll all pay dearly, both with our money and health. The economic drain caused by health issues associated with obesity is devastating. Today, we can barely bear the prices, let alone the estimated ten years from now.

What's On the Menu?

Are carbohydrates, protein, or fats making us fat? The bottom line is that you will gain weight if you eat too much of any or all of those nutrients. There's nothing special about low-carb diets, the glycemic index, or too much protein. Calories are what counts, and fad diets function (at least in the short term) as they minimize the overall quantity of calories you consume, easy and clear. The most convincing presentations at the summit advocated a diet high in complex carbohydrates, healthy fats, lean protein, and plenty of fruits and vegetables and discouraged processed carbs, sugars, trans fats, and saturated fats — just as we do at the WebMD Weight Loss Clinic.

No matter what else you consume, there's no such thing as a balanced diet without a big dose of produce — where you'll find over 1,000 health-promoting, disease-protective substances (antioxidants, phytochemicals, isoflavones, etc.), says Dean Ornish, MD.

The Blame Game

You could predict a decent amount of finger-pointing and allegations at a meeting with so many dietary heavy-hitters in attendance. But most agree that "the blame game" is a waste of energy and time. Obesity is a complicated issue and not the responsibility of any party, food, company, or advertisement. We need to help people take responsibility for what they eat instead of blaming each other, and inspire them to get some exercise. James O. Hill, Ph.D., Americaonthemove.org's co-founder, wants us all to put on pedometers and walk, walk, walk, add extra steps to our everyday lives in whatever way we can. Consolidate 10,000 stages for each day with a healthy diet, and you will be well on your way toward losing weight and improving your health.

One Size Does Not Fit All

Of this, the message is that there is no solution to the issue. Each of us needs to find a healthy eating plan that fits best for our lifestyles and build more healthy behaviors — like daily physical activity. It will contain lots of complex carbohydrates, fruits, vegetables, healthy fats, and lean protein, no matter which diet we adopt. And the amount of processed carbohydrates, trans-fats, and saturated fats should be reduced. Progress depends on how ready each of us is to commit to a healthier lifespan. We've discovered that weight management isn't just about education; most of us know that a healthy diet and daily exercise are the roads to better health. Now, we just need to do this — and get our friends, family, and neighbors to join us in fighting obesity.

Sirtuins and muscle fat

In the body, there is a family of genes that function as guardians of our muscle and, when under stress, avoid its breakdown: the sirtuins. SIRT1 is a strong Muscle Breakdown Inhibitor. So long, so SIRT1 is triggered, the muscle breakdown is prevented even when we are fasting, and we start burning fat for fuel. But SIRT1 's benefits aren't done with maintaining muscle mass. Sirtuins actually work to improve our skeletal muscle mass. We need to delve into the fascinating world of stem cells to understand how that process works. Our muscle contains a special form of stem cell, which is called a satellite cell that regulates its growth and regeneration.

Most of the time, satellite cells only sit there quietly, but they are stimulated when the muscle gets weakened or stressed. Via things like weight training, this is how our muscles get bigger. SIRT1 is important for activating satellite cells, and muscles are substantially weaker without their operation since they no longer have the capacity to properly grow or regenerate. However, we are giving a boost to our satellite cells by increasing SIRT1 activity, which encourages muscle growth and recovery.

Sirt foods VS Fasting

This leads us to a big question: if sirtuin activation increases muscle mass, then why do we lose muscle when we fast? After all, fasting activates our sirtuin genes as well. And herein lies one of the massive drawbacks of fasting.

This leads to a big question: if activation of the sirtuin increases muscle mass, why do we lose muscle when we fast? Fasting also stimulates our sirtuin genes, after all. And therein lies one of the fasting 's big drawbacks. Bear with us as we dig through the workings of this. Not all skeletal muscles are created equal to each other. We have two key forms, called type-1 and type-2 conveniently. Type-1 muscle is used for movements of longer length, while the type-2 muscle is used for brief bursts of more vigorous activity. And here's where it gets intriguing: fasting increases SIRT1 activity only in type-1 muscle fibers, not type-2. But type-1 muscle fiber size is preserved and even significantly increases when we fast.8 Unfortunately, in complete contrast to what happens in type-1 fibers during fasting, SIRT1 decreases rapidly in type-2 fibers. It means that fat burning slows down, and muscle breaks down to provide heat, instead.

But fasting for the muscles is a double-edged sword, with our type-2 fibers taking a hit. Type-2 fibers form the bulk of our concept of muscle. And even though our type-1 fiber mass is growing, with fasting, we also see a substantial overall loss of muscle. If we were able to avoid the breakdown, it would not only make us look aesthetically good but also help to encourage more loss of weight. And the way to do this is to combat the decrease in SIRT1 in muscle fiber type-2 that is caused by fasting. Researchers at Harvard Medical School tested this in an elegant mice study and found that the signals for muscle breakdown were turned off, and no muscle loss occurred by stimulating SIRT1 activity in type-2 fibers during fasting. The researchers then went a step further and tested the effects of increased SIRT1 activity on the muscle when the mice were fed rather than fasted, and found it stimulated very rapid growth of the muscle. In a week, muscle fibers with elevated levels of SIRT1 activity displayed an impressive weight gain of 20 percent.

Such results are very close to the outcome of our Sirtfood Diet trial, but in turn, our research has been milder. After increasing SIRT1 activity after consuming a diet rich in syrtfoods, most participants had no muscle loss — and for others, it was only a moderately strong, muscle mass that actually increased.

Chapter 4
TOP TWENTY SIRTFOODS DIETS

The list of the "top 20 sirtfoods" provided by the Sirtfood Diet includes;

1. Chilies
2. Strawberries
3. Turmeric
4. Walnuts
5. Buckwheat
6. Green Tea (Especially Matcha)
7. Kale
8. Arugula
9. Celery
10. Cocoa
11. Coffee
12. Red Endive
13. Red Onions
14. Extra Virgin Olive Oil
15. Garlic
16. Capers
17. Medjool Dates
18. Parsley
19. Red Wine
20. Soy

The diet combines sirtfoods and calorie restriction, both of which may trigger the body to produce higher levels of sirtuins. The creators of the diet claim that following the Diet will prompt quick weight reduction, while protecting you from chronic disease and maintaining muscle mass. Once you have completed the diet, you are encouraged to continue including sirtfoods and the diet's signature green juice into your regular diet.

Chilies

The chili has been an integral part of gastronomic experience worldwide for thousands of years. On one level, it's disconcerting that we'd be so enamored with it. Its pungent fire, caused by a substance called capsaicin in chilies, is designed as a mechanism of plant defense to cause pain and dissuade predators from feasting on it, and we appreciate that. The food and our infatuation with it are almost mysterious. Incredibly, one study found that consuming chilies together also enhances individual cooperation. And we know from a health perspective that their seductive heat is great to stimulate our sirtuins and improve our metabolism. The culinary applications of the chili are also endless, making it a simple way to offer a hefty Sirtfood boost to any dish. While we understand that not everyone is a fan of hot or spicy food, we hope we can entice you to consider adding small amounts of chilies, particularly in light of recent studies showing that those consuming spicy foods three or more times a week have a 14 percent lower death risk compared to those consuming them less than once a week. The hotter the chili, the stronger its Sirtfood credentials, but be careful and stick with what suits your own tastes. Serrano peppers are a great start- they tolerable for most people when packing heat, and for more experienced heat seekers, we suggest looking for Thai chilies for optimum sirtuin- activating benefits. They can be difficult to find in grocery stores but are mostly sold in specialty markets in Asia. Opt for deep-colored peppers, avoiding those with a wrinkled and fuzzy appearance.

Strawberries

In recent years, the fruit has been particularly vilified, getting a bad rap in the rising fervor toward sugar. Fortunately, such a malignant image couldn't be more undeserved for berry-lovers. While all berries are powerhouses of nutrition, strawberries are earning their top twenty Sirtfood status due to their abundance of the fisetin sirtuin activator. And now studies endorse daily eating strawberries to encourage healthy aging, keeping off Alzheimer's, cancer, diabetes, heart disease, and osteoporosis. It's very small as to their sugar content, a pure teaspoon of sugar per 3 / ounces. Amusingly, and naturally low in sugar itself, strawberries have marked effects on how the body treats carbohydrates. What researchers have found is that adding strawberries to carbohydrates decreases the need for insulin, effectively transforming the food into a constant energy releaser. Yet recent work also shows that eating strawberries in diabetes treatment has close results to the drug therapy. William Butler, the great physician of the seventeenth century, wrote in praise of the strawberry: "Doubtless God might have made a better berry, but without doubt He never did." We can only agree.

Turmeric

Turmeric, a cousin of ginger, is the new kid in food trends on the block, with Google naming it the ingredient of the 2015 breakout star. While we are only turning to it nowhere in the West, it has been valued for thousands of years in Asia, for both culinary and medical reasons. Incredibly, India is generating almost the entire world's turmeric supply, consuming 80% of it itself. In Asia, turmeric is used for treating skin disorders such as acne, psoriasis, dermatitis, and rash. Before Indian weddings, there is a ritual where the turmeric paste is applied as a skin beauty treatment to the bride and groom but also to symbolize the warding off evil. One factor that limits turmeric 's effectiveness is that the main sirtuin-activating compound, curcumin, is poorly absorbed by the body as we consume it. Analysis, however, shows that we can solve this by boiling it in oil, adding fat, and adding black pepper, all of which increase its absorption dramatically.

This suits well with traditional Indian cuisine, wherei n curries and other hot dishes it is traditionally mixed with ghee and black pepper, and again prove that scie nce just catches up with the age-
old wisdom of traditional eating methods.

Walnuts

Dating back to 7000 BCE, walnuts are the oldest known tree food, originating in ancient Persia, where they were the preserve of royalty. Fast-forward to today, and walnuts are a success story for the United States. California is leading the way, with California's Central Valley famous for being the prime walnut-growing area. California walnuts provide the United States with 99% of commercial supply and whopping three-quarters of worldwide walnut trade. Walnuts lead the way as the number one nut for health, according to the NuVal system, which ranks foods according to how safe they are and has been endorsed by the American College of Preventive Medicine. But what really makes walnuts stand out for us is how they fly in the face of traditional thinking: they are high in fat and calories, but well-established for weight loss and the risk of metabolic diseases like cardiovascular disease and diabetes is reduced. That is the strength of triggering the sirtuin. The recent research showing walnuts to be an effective anti-aging food is less well known but equally fascinating. Research also points to their benefits as a brain food with the potential to slow down brain aging and reduce the risk of degenerative brain disorders, as well as preventing the decline in physical function with age.

Buckwheat

Buckwheat was one of Japan's first domesticated crops, and the story goes that when Buddhist monks made long trips into the mountains, they 'd only bring a cooking pot and a buckwheat bag for food. Buckwheat is so nutritious that this was all they wanted, and it kept them up for weeks. We 're big fans of buckwheat too. Firstly, since it is one of a sirtuin activator's best-known outlets, named rutin. But also because it has advantages as a cover crop, improving soil quality and suppressing weed growth, making it a great crop for environmentally friendly and sustainable agriculture. One reason buckwheat is head and shoulders above other, more popular grains is possible because it's not a grain at all — it's actually a rhubarb-related fruit seed. Having one of the highest protein content of any grain, as well as being a Sirtfood powerhouse, makes it an unrivaled alternative to more widely used grains. However, it is as flexible as any grain, and being naturally gluten-free, it is a perfect alternative for those intolerant to gluten.

Green Tea (Especially Matcha)

Many will be familiar with green tea, the toast of the Orient, and ever more popular in the West. With the rising awareness of its health benefits, green tea consumption is related to less cancer, heart disease, diabetes, and osteoporosis. The reason it is thought that green tea is so good for us is primarily due to its rich content of a group of powerful plant compounds called catechins, the star of the show being a particular type of sirtuin-activating catechin known as epigallocatechin gallate (EGCG). But what the fuss about matcha is all about? We like to think of matcha on the steroids as normal green tea. In comparison to traditional green tea, which is prepared as an infusion, it is a special powdered green tea which is prepared by dissolving directly in water. The upshot of drinking matcha is that it contains significantly higher levels of the sirtuin-activating compound EGCG than other green tea forms. Zen priests describe matcha as the "ultimate mental and medical remedy [which] has the potential to make one 's life more full" if you are looking for more endorsement.

Kale

We are at heart cynics, so we are always skeptical about what drives the latest craze for superfood advertising. Was it science, or is it interests at stake? In recent years few foods have exploded as dramatically as kale on the health scene. Described as the "lean, green brassica queen" (referring to its cruciferous vegetable family), it has become the chic vegetable for which all health-lovers and foodies are gunning. Every October, there is also a National Day of the Kale. But you don't have to wait until then to show your kale pride: there are T-shirts too, with trendy slogans such as "Powered by Kale" and "Highway to Kale." That's enough for us to set the alarm bells ringing. We've done the research, filled with suspicions, and we have to admit that our conclusion is that kale really deserves her pleasures (although we still don't recommend the T-shirts!). The reason we 're pro-kale is that it boasts bumper quantities of the quercetin and kaempferol sirtuin-activating nutrients, making it a must-include in the Sirtfood Diet and the foundation of our green Sirtfood juice. What's so exciting about kale is that kale is available anywhere, locally produced, and very inexpensive, unlike the typical expensive, hard-to-source, and exorbitantly priced so-called superfoods!

Arugula

Clearly, Arugula (also known as rocket, rucola, rugula, and roquette) has a colorful background in American food culture. A pungent green salad leaf with a distinctive peppery taste, it rapidly ascended from humble origins as the basis of many Mediterranean peasant dishes to become a symbol of food snobbery in the United States, also contributing to the coining of the word arugulance!

But long before it was a salad leaf wielded in a class war, arugula was revered by the ancient Greeks and Romans for its medicinal properties. Commonly used as a diuretic and digestive aid, it gained its true fame from its reputation for having potent aphrodisiac properties, so much so that growth of arugula was banned in monasteries in the Middle Ages, and the famous Roman poet Virgil wrote that "the rocket excites the sexual desire of drowsy people." However, what really excites us about arugula is its bumper quantities of the sirtuin-activating kaempferol and quercetin nutrients. A combination of kaempferol and quercetin is being investigated as a cosmetic ingredient in addition to powerful sirtuin-activating properties because together, they moisturize and enhance collagen synthesis in the skin. With those credentials, it's time to remove that elitist tag and make this the leaf of choice for salad bases, where it beautifully pairs with an extra virgin olive oil dressing, combining to create a strong double act of Sirtfood.

Celery

For centuries, Celery was around and revered — with leaves found adorning the remains of the Egyptian pharaoh Tutankhamun who died around 1323 BCE. Early strains were very bitter, and celery was generally considered a medicinal plant for cleaning and detoxification to prevent disease. This is particularly interesting considering that liver, kidney, and gut safety are among the many promising benefits that science is now showing.

It was domesticated as a vegetable in the seventeenth century, and selective breeding diminished its strong bitter flavor in favor of sweeter varieties, thus establishing its place as a traditional salad vegetable. It is important to remember when it comes to celery, that there are two types: blanched/yellow and Pascal / green. Blanching is a technique developed to reduce the characteristic bitter taste of the celery, which has been considered to be too intense.

It involves shading the celery before harvesting from sunshine, resulting in a paler color and a milder flavor. What a travesty that is, for blanching dumbs down the sirtuin-activating properties of celery as well as dumbing down the flavor. Thankfully, the tide is shifting, and people are demanding true and distinct flavor, moving back to the greener variety. Green celery is the sort that we suggest you use in both the green juices and meals, with the heart and leaves being the most nutritious pieces.

Cocoa

It's no surprise to learn that cocoa was considered a sacred food for ancient civilizations like the Aztecs and Mayans, and was usually reserved for the elite and warriors, served at feasts to gain loyalty and duty. Indeed, there was such high regard for the cocoa bean that it was even used as a form of currency. It was usually served as a frothy beverage back then. But what could be a more delicious way to get our dietary amount of cacao than by chocolate? Unfortunately, there's no count here for the diluted, refined, and highly sweetened milk chocolate we commonly munch. We 're talking about chocolate with 85 percent solids of cocoa to earn the Sirtfood badge. But even then, apart from the percentage of cocoa, not all chocolate is produced equal. To its acidity and give it a darker color, chocolate is often treated with an alkalizing agent (known as the Dutch process).

Sadly, this process diminishes its sirtuin-activating flavanols significantly, thus seriously compromising its health-promoting content. Fortunately, and unlike in several other nations, food labeling laws in the United States allow alkalized cocoa to be reported as such and labeled "alkali processed." We suggest avoiding such items, even though they advertise a higher percentage of cocoa, and opting instead for those who have not undergone Dutch processing to enjoy the true benefits of cocoa.

Coffee

What's all that about Sirtfood Coffee? We 're listening to you. We can assure you that this is no typo. Gone are the days when a twinge of remorse had to balance our enjoyment of coffee. The work is unambiguous: coffee is a bona fide food for wellbeing. Indeed it is a true treasure chest of fantastic nutrients that trigger sirtuin. And with more than half of Americans consuming coffee every day (to the tune of $40 billion a year!), coffee enjoys the accolade of becoming America's number one source of polyphenols. The biggest irony is that the one thing we were chastised by so many fitness "experts" for doing was, in reality, the best thing we were doing for our wellbeing each day. This is why coffee drinkers have significantly less diabetes and lower rates of some cancers and neurodegenerative disease. As for the ultimate irony, coffee, rather than being a poison, actually protects our livers and makes them healthier! And contrary to the common misconception that coffee dehydrates the body, it is now well known not to be the case, with coffee (and tea) contributing very well to daily coffee drinkers' fluid intake. And while we understand that coffee is not for everyone and some people might be very susceptible to the effects of caffeine, it's happy days for those who love a cup of joe.

Red Endive

Endive is a fairly new kid on the block in so far as vegetables go. Legend has it that a Belgian farmer found endive in 1830, by mistake. The farmer stored chicory roots in his cellar, and then used them as a type of coffee substitute, only to forget them. Upon his return, he discovered that white leaves had sprouted, which he found to be tender, crunchy, and rather delicious upon degustation. Endive is now grown all over the world, including the USA, and earns its Sirtfood badge thanks to its impressive sirtuin activator luteolin content. And besides the proven sirtuin-activating benefits, luteolin intake has become a promising approach to therapy to enhance sociability in autistic children. It has a crisp texture and a sweet taste for those new to endive, followed by a gentle and friendly bitterness. If you're ever stuck on how to increase endive in your diet, you can't fail by adding her leaves to a salad where her warm, tart flavor adds the perfect bite to an extra virgin olive oil dressing based on zesty. Red is best, just like an onion, but the yellow variety can also be considered a Sirtfood. So while the red variety may sometimes be more difficult to find, you can rest assured that yellow is a perfectly appropriate alternative.

Red Onions

Since the time of our prehistoric predecessors, onions have been a dietary staple, being one of the earliest crops to be cultivated, some 5,000 years ago. With such a long history of use and such potent health-giving properties, many cultures that came before us have revered onions. They were held especially by the Egyptians as objects of worship, regarding their circle-within-a-circle structure as symbolic of eternal life. And the Greeks claimed that onions made athletes stronger. Athletes will eat their way through large quantities of oignons before the Olympic Games, even drinking the water! It's an amazing testament to how important ancient culinary knowledge can be when we remember that onions deserve their top twenty Sirtfood status because they're chock-full of the sirtuin-activating compound quercetin — the very compound that the sports science community has recently started aggressively researching and promoting to boost sports performance. And why the red ones? Simply because they have the highest content of quercetin, although the regular yellow ones do not lag too far behind, and are also a good inclusion.

Extra Virgin Olive Oil

Olive oil is the most renowned of Mediterranean traditional diets. The olive tree is among the world's oldest-known cultivated plants, also known as the "immortal tree." And since people started squeezing olives in stone mortars to gather them, the oil has been respected, almost 7,000 years ago. Hippocrates cited it as a cure-all; now, a few decades later, modern science confidently claims its wonderful health benefits.

There is now a wealth of scientific data showing that regular olive oil consumption is highly cardioprotective, as well as playing a role in reducing the risk of major modern-day diseases such as diabetes, certain cancers, and osteoporosis, and associated with increased longevity. There is now a wealth of scientific data showing that regular olive oil consumption is highly cardioprotective, as well as playing a role in reducing the risk of major modern-day diseases such as diabetes, certain cancers, and osteoporosis, and associated with increased longevity.

Garlic

Garlic has been considered one of Nature's wonder foods for thousands of years, with soothing and rejuvenating properties. Egyptians fed pyramid workers with garlic to enhance their immunity, avoid various diseases, and strengthen their performance through their ability to resist fatigue. Garlic is a potent natural antibiotic and antifungal that is sometimes used to help cure ulcers in the stomach. By speeding the elimination of waste products from the body, it can stimulate the lymphatic system to "detox." And as well as being investigated for fat loss, it also packs a potent heart health punch, lowering cholesterol by about 10 percent, and lowering blood pressure by 5 to 7 percent, as well as lowering blood stickiness and blood sugar levels.7 And if you're worried about the off-putting garlic odor, note. When women were asked to assess a selection of men's body odors, those men who ingested four or more garlic cloves a day were found to have a much more attractive and friendly odor. Researchers suggest this is because it is viewed as signaling better health. And there's always mints for the fresher breath, of course! Eating garlic has a trick to get full profit. In garlic, the Sirtfood nutrients are complemented by another key nutrient in it called allicin, which gives off the characteristic aroma of garlic. But after physical "injury" to the bulb, allicin only forms in garlic. And, when exposed to heat (cooking) or low pH (stomach acid), its formation is halted. So when preparing garlic, chop, thin, or crush, and then allow it to sit for about ten minutes before cooking or eating the allicin.

Capers

In case you 're not so familiar with capers, we 're talking about those salty, dark green, pellet-like things on top of a pizza that you may only have had occasion to see. But certainly, they are one of the most undervalued and neglected foods out there. Intriguingly, they are actually the caper bush's flower buds, which grow abundantly in the Mediterranean before being picked and preserved by hand. Studies now show that capers possess important antimicrobial, antidiabetic, anti-inflammatory, immunomodulatory, and antiviral properties and have a rich history of being used as a medicine in the Mediterranean and North Africa. Hardly surprising when we discover that they are crammed full of sirtuin-activating nutrients. We think it is about time these tiny morsels got their share of glory, too often overshadowed by the other big hitters from the Mediterranean diet. Flavor-wise it's a case of big stuff coming in small packages, as they're sure they 're punching. Yet if you don't know how to use them, then don't feel scared. For these diminutive nutrient superstars, when paired with the right ingredients, have a wonderfully distinctive and inimitable sour/salty taste to round off a dish in style, we'll soon have you up to speed and falling head over heels.

Medjool Dates

It comes as a surprise to include Medjool dates in a list of foods that stimulate weight loss and promote health—especially when we tell you that Medjool dates contain a staggering 66 percent sugar. Sugar doesn't have any sirtuin-activating properties at all; rather, it has well-established links to obesity, heart disease, and diabetes — just the opposite of what we're looking to achieve. Yet processed and refined sugar is very different from sugar borne in a naturally supplied vehicle filled with sirtuin-activating polyphenols: the date of the Medjool. Medjool dates, consumed in moderation, do not really have any real significant blood-sugar-raising effects, in complete contrast with regular sugar. Instead, eating them is associated with developing less diabetes and heart disease. They have been a staple food worldwide for centuries, and there has been an explosion of scientific interest in dates in recent years, which sees them emerging as a potential medicine for a number of diseases. Herein lies the uniqueness and power of the Sirtfood Diet: it refutes the dogma and allows you to indulge in sweet things in moderation without feeling guilty.

Parsley

Parsley is a food conundrum. It appears so often in recipes, and so often it's the token green man. At best, we serve a couple of chopped sprigs and tossed as an afterthought on a meal, at worst a single sprig for decorative purposes only. That way, there on the plate, it is always languishing long after we have finished eating. This culinary style stems from its common use in ancient Rome as a garnish for eating after meals in order to refresh breath, rather than being part of the meal itself. And what a shame, because parsley is a wonderful food that packs a vivid, refreshing taste full of character. Taste aside, what makes parsley very unique is that it is an excellent source of the sirtuin-activating nutrient apigenin, a real blessing because it is rarely contained in other foods in large amounts. In our brains, apigenin binds fascinatingly to the benzodiazepine receptors, helping us to relax and help us to sleep. Stack it all up, and it's time we appreciated parsley not as omnipresent food confetti, but as a food in its own right to reap the wonderful health benefits that it can offer.

Red Wine

Any list of the top twenty Sirtfoods will not be complete without the inclusion of the original Sirtfood, red wine. The French phenomenon made headlines in the early 1990s, with it being discovered that despite the French appearing to do something wrong when it came to health (smoking, lack of exercise, and rich food consumption), they had lower death rates from heart disease than countries like the United States. The explanation for this was suggested by doctors was the copious amount of red wine drank. Danish researchers then published work in 1995 to show that low-to - moderate consumption of red wine decreased death rates, while comparable levels of beer alcohol had no effect, and comparable intakes of hard liquors increased death rates. Obviously, in 2003, the rich quality of red wine from a bevy of sirtuin-activating nutrients was discovered, and the rest, as they claim, was made history. But there is much more to the outstanding resume of red wine. Red wine seems to be able to stop the common cold, with moderate wine drinkers seeing a reduction in its incidence of more than 40%.12 Studies also show benefits for oral health and cavity prevention.13 With moderate consumption, social interaction and out-of-the-box thinking have also been shown to increase the after-work drink between cavities. It appears that colleagues debating work ventures have roots in solid research. Moderation is, of course, important. To gain from this, only small quantities are required, and excess alcohol quickly undoes the good. The sweet spot seems to stick up to one 5-ounce drink per day for women and up to two 5-ounce drinks per day for men according to US guidelines. Wines from the New York region (especially pinot noir, cabernet sauvignon, and merlot) have the highest polyphenol content of the most widely available wines to ensure maximum sirtuin-activating bang for your buck.

Soy

Soy products have a long history as an integral part of the diet of many countries in Asia-Pacific, such as China, Japan, and Korea. Researchers first turned on to soy after discovering that high soy-consuming countries had significantly lower rates of certain cancers, especially breast and prostate cancers. It is believed to be attributed to a specific category of polyphenols in soybeans known as isoflavones, which can favorably affect how estrogens function in the body, like daidzein and formononetin sirtuin-activators. Soy product intake has also been related to a decrease in the incidence or severity of a number of conditions such as cardiovascular disease, effects of menopause, and bone loss. Highly refined, nutrient-stripped soybean types are now a common component applied to various packaged foods. The benefits are only reaped from natural soy products such as tofu, an excellent vegan protein source, or in a fermented form such as tempeh, natto, or our favorite, miso, a typical Japanese paste fermented with a naturally occurring fungus that results in an intense umami taste.

Chapter 5
APPLICATION SIRTFOOD DIET PLANS

Eating some quality foods will improve the pathways of your "skinny gene" and allow you to shed some unnecessary weight in seven days. Food like kale, dark chocolate, and wine has a natural compound known as polyphenols that looks like fitness workout results and fasting. Strawberries, cinnamon, and turmeric are also powerful sirt-foods. These foods can activate the steps or potentials of the sirtuin to help promote weight loss.

There are 2 phases to follow the sirtfood diet:

Phase 1 Of The Sirtfood Diet

Calorie consumption is constrained to 1,000 calories in the initial three days (that is more than on a 5:2 day of fasting). The diet consists of 3 Sirtfood-full green juices and 1 Sirtfood-filled meal and two dark chocolate servings.

For the remaining four-day calories intake should be raised to 1,500 calories, and two sirtfood-filled green juices and two sirtfood-rich meals should be included daily in the diet. You are not allowed to drink any alcohol in the early "Phase 1 stage," but you are free to take water and green tea.

Phase 2 Of The Sirtfood Diet

Phase 2 is not for reducing calorie consumption. Daily consumption includes 3 Sirtfood-rich foods and one green juice, and if possible, the alternative of 1 or 2 Sirtfood crunch snacks. You are permitted to take red wine in the second phase 2 but not too much (they encourage you to take 2-3 glasses of red wine weekly), as well as soda, tea, coffee, and green tea too.

PHASES OF THE SIRTFOOD DIET

There are two phases for this diet; Phase 1 and Phase2

Phase 1: 7 pounds in seven days

Monday: three green juices

Breakfast: water + tea or espresso + a cup of green juice;

Lunch: green juice

Snack: a square of dark chocolate;

Dinner: Sirt meal

After dinner: a square of dark chocolate.

Drink the juices at three different times of the day (for instance, in the morning as soon as you wake, mid-morning and mid-afternoon) and choose the usual or vegan dish: pan-fried oriental prawns with buckwheat spaghetti or miso and tofu with sesame glaze and sautéed vegetables (vegan dish).

Tuesday: 3 green juices

Breakfast: water + tea or espresso + a cup of green juice

Lunch: 2 green juices before dinner;

Snack: a square of dark chocolate;

Dinner: Sirt meal

After dinner: a square of dark chocolate.

Welcome to Sirtfood Diet day 2. The formula is similar to that of the first day, and only the solid meal varies. You'll have dark chocolate today, too, and the same will be true for tomorrow. This food is so amazing we don't need an excuse to eat it.

Chocolate must be at least 85% cocoa to receive the title of a "Sirt chocolate." And even with that percentage of the various types of chocolate, not all of them are the same. This substance is also treated with an alkalizing agent (the so-called "Netherlands process") to reduce its acidity and give it a darker color. Unfortunately, this process greatly reduces the activation of sirtuins by flavonoids, compromising their health benefits. Lindt Excellence 85% chocolate, is not subject to the process in the Netherlands and is therefore often recommended.

The menu also includes capers on day 2, as well. They are not fruits, despite what many may think, but buds that grow in Mediterranean countries and are picked by hand. They are great Sirt foods because they are very nutrient-rich And quercetin and kaempferol. From the flavor standpoint, they are tiny taste concentrates. If you have never used them, feel no intimidation. You will see, if combined with the right ingredients, they will taste amazing and will give your dishes an unmistakable and inimitable aroma.

You must consume on the second day: 3 green Sirt juices and one strong (normal or vegan) meal. Drink the juices at three distinct times of the day (for example, when you wake up in the morning, mid-morning and mid-afternoon) and pick either the usual or vegan dish: turkey with capers, parsley and sage on spicy couscous or curly couscous cauliflower and buckwheat red onion Dahl (vegan dish)

Wednesday: 3 green juices

Breakfast: water + tea or espresso + a cup of green juice

Lunch: 2 green juices before dinner;

Snack: a square of dark chocolate;

Dinner: Sirt meal

After dinner: a square of dark chocolate.

You are now on the third day, and even though the style is again similar to that of days 1 and 2, then the time has come to spice it with a basic ingredient. Chili has been a fundamental element of the worldwide gastronomic experiences for thousands of years. As for the health effects, we've already seen that its spiciness is perfect to activate sirtuins and stimulate metabolism. Chili's applications are endless and thus provide a simple way to eat a daily Sirt meal.

If you're not a big chili expert, we recommend the Bird 's Eye (sometimes called Thai chili), because, for sirtuins, it's the best. This is the last day you consume three green juices a day; you switch to two tomorrow. And we take this opportunity to browse other beverages you may have during your diet. We all know that green tea is good for health and water is very good, of course, but what about coffee? More than half of people drink at least one coffee a day, but still with a hint of shame because others claiming it's a crime and an unhealthy habit. Studies show that coffee is a true treasure trove of beneficial plant substances. That's why coffee drinkers are the least likely to get diabetes, certain forms of cancer, and neurodegenerative diseases. In addition, coffee isn't just a toxin; it protects the liver and makes it even healthier!

You will ingest three green Sirt juices and one solid meal on the third day (normal or vegan, see below). Drink the juices at three different times of the day (e.g., in the morning as soon as you wake up, mid-morning and mid-afternoon) and pick the usual or vegan dish: aromatic chicken breast with kale, red onion, tomato sauce, and chili or baked tofu with harissa on spicy couscous (vegan platter)

Thursday: 2 green juices

Breakfast: water + tea or espresso + a cup of green juice;

Lunch: Sirt food;

Snack: 1 green juice before dinner

Dinner: Sirt food

The Sirtfood Diet's fourth day has arrived, and you are halfway through your journey into a leaner, healthier body. The big change from the previous three days is you're only going to drink two juices instead of three and you're going to have two solid

60

meals in place of one. That means you'll have two green juices and two strong meals on the fourth day and the next day, all delicious and rich in Sirt foods. It may seem surprising to include Medjoul dates in a list of foods that support weight loss and good health. Especially if you think they have 66 percent sugar in them. Sugar does not have any stimulating properties against sirtuins. On the contrary, it has well-known linkages with obesity, heart disease, and diabetes; in short, we target only at the antipodes of the targets. But industrially refined and processed sugar in food, which also contains sirtuin-activating polyphenols is very different from the sugar present: the Medjoul dates. These dates, consumed in moderation, do not increase blood glucose levels as opposed to normal sugar.

You must intake on the fourth day: 2 green Sirt juices, two solid meals (normal or vegan) Drink the juices at various times of the day (for example the first in the morning as soon as you wake up or in the middle of the morning, the second in the middle of the afternoon) and select the normal or vegan dishes: muesli sirt, pan-fried salmon filet with caramelized chicory, rocket salad and celery leaves or muesli Sirt and Tuscan stewed beans (vegan dish)

Friday: 2 green juices

Breakfast: water + tea or espresso + a cup of green juice

Lunch: Sirt food

Snack: a green juice before dinner;

Dinner: Sirt food

You have hit the fifth day, so it's time to add some berries. Because of its high sugar content, the fruit was the subject of the bad advertisement. That is not applicable to berries. The sugar content of strawberries is very low: one teaspoon per 100 grams. They also have an excellent influence on how simple sugars are processed in the body. Scientists have found that this causes a reduction in insulin demand if we add strawberries to simple sugars, and thus transforms food into a machine that releases energy for a long time to come. Therefore strawberries are a perfect diet element that will help you lose weight and get back into shape. They are also delicious and extremely versatile, as you'll discover the fresh and light Middle Eastern tabbouleh in the Sirt version.

The Miso is a popular Japanese soup made from fermented soy. Miso has a powerful scent of umami, a complete explosion for the taste buds. We know better the monosodium glutamate in our modern society, produced artificially to replicate the same taste. Needless to say, deriving the magical umami taste from conventional and natural ingredients, full of beneficial substances, is much more preferable. It is found in all good supermarkets and healthy food stores in the form of a paste and should be present in each kitchen to give many different dishes a touch of taste.

Because umami flavors enhance one another, miso is perfectly associated with other tasty / umami foods, particularly when it comes to cooked proteins, as you will discover in the very tasty, quick, and easy dishes you are going to eat today. You will ingest two green Sirt juices and two solid (normal or vegan) meals on the fifth day. Drink the juices at various times of the day (for instance; the first in the middle of the morning or as soon as you wake up; the second in the middle of the afternoon) and pick the usual or vegan dishes: buckwheat Tabbouleh with strawberries, baked cod marinated in miso with sautéed. Sesame or buckwheat vegetables and strawberry Tabbouleh (vegan platter) and kale (vegan dish).

Saturday: 2 green juices

Breakfast: water + tea or espresso + a cup of green juice

Lunch: Sirt food

Snack: a green juice before dinner;

Dinner: Sirt food

There is no better Sirt food than olive oil and red wine. Virgin olive oil is only obtained by mechanical means from the fruit, in conditions that do not deteriorate it, so you can be sure of its quality and polyphenol content. "Extra virgin" oil is the first pressing oil ("virgin" is the product of the second pressing) and thus has more flavor and higher quality: this is what we highly prefer to use while cooking.

No Sirt menu would be complete without red wine, which is one of the diet's cornerstones. It contains resveratrol and piceatannol sirtuins activators that are likely to explain the longevity and slenderness associated with the traditional French way of life and that are at the root of the enthusiasm unleashed by Sirt foods. You'll expect two green Sirt juices and two strong (normal or vegan) meals on the sixth day.

Drink the juices at different times of the day (for example, the first in the middle of the morning or as soon as you wake up, the second in the middle of the afternoon) and choose the ordinary or vegan dishes: Super Sirt salad and grilled beef fillet with red wine sauce, onion rings, curly garlic kale and roasted potatoes with aromatic herbs, or Super lentil Sirt salad (vegan dish) and red bean mole sauce with roasted potato (vegan dish).

Sunday: 2 green juices

Breakfast: a bowl of Sirt Muesli + a cup of green juice

Lunch: Sirt food

Snack: a cup of green juice;

Dinner: Sirt food

The seventh day is the final of the diet's step 1. Instead of seeing it as an end, see it as a beginning, for you are about to embark on a new life in which sirt foods can play a central role in your diet. Today's menu is a perfect example of how easy it is to integrate them into your daily diet in abundance. Just take your favorite dishes, and turn them into a Sirt banquet with a pinch of imagination. Walnuts are perfect Sirt food because they refute current views. They have high-fat content and many calories, yet they have been shown to contribute to weight reduction and metabolic diseases, all thanks to sirtuin activation. Also, they are a versatile ingredient, excellent in baked dishes, salads, and alone as a snack.

We can apply the same reasoning to a dish that is easy to prepare, such as an omelet. The dish must be the traditional recipe that the whole family appreciates, and it must be easy to turn into a Sirt dish with a few little tricks. We use bacon in our recycling. Why? For what? Just because it just fits perfectly. The Sirtfood Diet tells us what to include, not what to exclude, and this allows us to change our eating habits over the long term. Isn't that, after all, the secret of not getting the lost pounds back and staying healthy?

You'll assume two green Sirt juices on the seventh day; 2 solid (normal or vegan) meals. Drink the juices at different times of the day (for example the first in the morning as soon as you wake up or in the middle of the morning, the second in the middle of the afternoon) and choose the normal or vegan dishes: omelet sirt and boiled aubergine wedges with walnut and parsley pesto and tomato salad (vegan dish).

There are no calorie restrictions during the second phase but indications on which Sirt foods should be eaten to consolidate weight loss and not run the risk of getting the kilograms lost back.

Phase 2: Maintenance

Congratulations, You have finished the first "hardcore" week. The second step is the simpler one and is the actual integration of food choices loaded with sirtuin into your daily diet or meals. You can call this the "stage of maintenance." Your body will be subjected to the fat-burning level, and muscle gain plus a boost to your immune system and overall health. You can now get three healthy SirtFood-filled meals per day for this process plus one green juice per day.

There is no "dieting" but more about selecting safer alternatives with as much as possible, adding SirtFood to every meal. I will be providing some SirtFood inclusive recipes for tasty dishes to give you an idea of how exciting and healthy this diet journey is. Now you are going back to a daily intake of calories with the intention of keeping your weight loss stable and your Sirtfood intake high. By now, you should have undergone a degree of weight loss, but you should still feel trimming and revitalizing.

Phase 2 lasts for 14 days. During this time you will eat three sirtfood-rich meals, one sirtfood-green juice and up to 2 optional snacks of Sirtfood bite. Strict calorie-counting is actively discouraged if you follow recommendations and eat reasonable portions of balanced meals; you shouldn't feel hungry or consume too much. You will have the same drinks you drank in step 1. With the small improvement, you 're welcome to enjoy the occasional glass of red wine (though you don't drink more than three a week).

Chapter 6
SIRTFOOD DIET AND EXERCISE

Joining diet and nutrition with The Sirtfood diet

With 52 percent of Americans agreeing that they think it's easier to do their charges than to see how to eat consistently, it's important to present a form of eating that transforms into a lifestyle as opposed to a coincidental prevailing fashion diet. It might not be that hard for those of us to get smaller or keep a solid weight, but the Sirtfood diet will benefit the fighting individuals. Be that as it may, something shouldn't be said about starting the Sirtfood diet with work out, is it appropriate to stay away from exercise altogether or pose it once you've begun the diet?

The principles of the Sirt Diet

With an estimated 650 million heavy grown-ups worldwide, it's vital to discover feasible smart diet and exercise schemes, don't refuse you anything you want, and don't expect you to exercise all week. The diet Sirtfood does exactly that. The idea is that sure nourishments can provide dynamic the pathways of 'thin consistency' that are usually triggered by fasting and exercise. Luckily other foods and beverages, including bland chocolate and red wine, produce synthetic substances called polyphenols that enact the qualities that duplicate the operation and fasting impacts.

Exercise during the first few weeks

Although your body adjusts to less calories, it is natural to quit or lessen the exercise during the first week or second of the diet, when your calorie intake is decreased. Tune in to your body, and don't find out if you feel tired or have less energy than expected. Rather ensure you stay focused on the rules that apply to a solid lifestyle, including, for example, satisfactory day-to-day levels of soil fiber, protein, and products.

Chapter 7
FREQUENTLY ASKED QUESTIONS

Q. Does The Sirtfood Diet Work?

Indeed, it does as indicated by their numerous celebrity endorsements. The subsequent book was endorsed by David Haye (Heavyweight Boxer), Jodie Kidd (Model), Sir Ben Ainslie (Olympic Gold Medallist), Lorraine Pascale (TV Chef and Food Writer), and an entire load of other superstars who all claim that the Sirtfood Diet has helped them get thinner, form muscle and look and feel extraordinary. Though my preferred endorsement is certainly the one which is just ascribed to a wife of a participant and which reads 'Thank you! My better half is looking extra hot.'

Q. Who came up with the Sirtfood Diet?

Two authors and wellbeing specialists known as Glen Matten and Aidan Goggins, whose spotlight has consistently been on healthy dieting as opposed to weight reduction. In their new book The Sirtfood Diet, the pair spread out a feast plan which includes consuming three sirtfood green juices a day joined by adjusted sirtfood-rich suppers, for example, 'buckwheat and prawn pan sear' or 'smoked salmon sirt super sala

Q. Can you lose weight on the diet?

The Sirtfood Diet incorporates numerous nutritious foods that are valuable for weight reduction, for example, celery, kale, lean red meat, green tea, lean chicken, and parsley, and Medjool dates, says Dr. Apovian. The diet additionally limits or eliminates numerous nourishments that are known to cause weight increase, for example, refined flours, added sugars, and processed foods with next to zero dietary benefits. And thanks to that strangely low-calorie consumption, followers will probably shed pounds provided they stay on course.

Q. What happens after you are done with the sirt food diet?

This Diet isn't intended to be an erratic 'diet' but rather a lifestyle. You are encouraged when you've finished the initial three weeks, to keep eating a diet rich in Sirtfoods, and to continue drinking your green juice every day. The creators of The

Sirtfood Diet recommend that Phases 1 and 2 can be rehashed as and when fundamental for a health boost, or if things have gone somewhat off track.

Q. What foods are high in sirtuins?

This book contains a rundown of the main 20 nourishments that are high in sirtuins (chapter 4), which sounds more like a trending food list than another, advanced diet. Models include arugula, Medjool dates, red wine, chilies, espresso, green tea, turmeric, pecans, and the wellbeing cognizant top favorite-kale. Dr. Youdim takes note of that while the nourishments being promoted are healthy, they won't really promote weight reduction on their own.

Q. What are the benefits?

You will lose weight if you follow this diet intently. "Regardless of whether you're eating 1,000 calories of tacos, or 1,000 calories of snickerdoodles, 1,000 calories of kale, you will shed pounds at 1,000 calories!" says Dr. Youdim.

The benefits of Sirtfood also include the following;

Drive your weight loss from fat and not muscle;

Ensure you look better, feel better and have more energy;

Prepare your body for long-term weight loss success;

Stop you having to experience severe fasting or acute hunger;

Free you from exhausting exercise sessions;

Be a springboard for a longer, healthier and disease-free life.

CONCLUSION

What seems like a snack lifted directly from a science fiction movie, a 'sirtfood' is really a food high in sirtuin activators. Sirtuins are a kind of protein that shields the cells in our bodies from dying or getting inflamed through illness; however, research has additionally shown that they can help control your digestion, burn fat and increase muscle. Hence, the new 'wonder food' tag. "Sirtfood" seems like something created by aliens, brought to earth for human consumption with the expectation of gaining world domination and mind control. In fact, Sirt foods are basically foods high in sirtuins. Uh, come back again? Sirtuins are a kind of protein that studies on fruit flies and mice have indicated direct digestion, burn fat, increase muscle mass.

The Sirtfood Diet book was first distributed in the U.K. in 2016. But, the United States release of the book has sparked more interest in the arrangement. The diet started getting publicity when Adele debuted her slimmer figure at the Billboard Music Awards last May. Her trainer, Pete Geracimo, is a colossal fanatic of the diet and says the singer shed thirty pounds from following a Sirt food diet. (Here, Adele gets genuine about getting healthy.)

As indicated by the book, this plan can assist you with burning fat and boost your vitality, preparing your body for long haul weight reduction achievement, and a more healthy, disease-free life and all that while drinking red wine. Sounds like practically the ideal diet, isn't that so? All things considered, before you burn through your funds, stocking up on sirtuins-filled fixings, know the pros and cons.

Good Luck!

SIRT FOOD RECIPES

Sirt Green Juice

Total Calories: 1,000

Ingredients:

2 big handfuls kale (75 g); Very small lovage leaves (5g) (optional); 2 to 3 large celery stalks (150 g) including leaves1/2 green apple.; 1/2-Lemon juice; 1/2 tablespoon matcha green tea; a large handful (30g) rocket ; a very small handful (5g) flat-leaf parsley

Instructions:

Mix greens (rocket, parsley, lovage and kale, if used) together, then make a juice. Juicers can vary in their performance when making juice of leafy green veggies, and you'll need to rejuice the remains before you move further to some other ingredients. So, the aim is to make 50ml juice that is extracted from the green vegges.

Now make juice of apple and celery.

You can also peel off the lemon and place it in the juicer, but it's easier to crush the lemon juice by hand. You must have about 250ml juice by this stage, possibly slightly more. Just after the juice is blended and prepared to drink, add the green tea matcha. Pour a little juice in a glass, add matcha and mix with a teaspoon. We just used matcha only first two drinks in a day because it includes small levels of caffeine (as there is the same quality as a regular tea cup). It can keep people awake if they're drunk late. When matcha is dissolved, you can add the rest of juice. Give a quick and final swirl, and then drink your tea. Top it up with water to add flavor.

Melon Juice And Grape

Total Calories: 125 - Serves for 1 - Preparation time: 2 minutes

Ingredients:

½ cucumbers peel it if needed, cut half, remove the seeds and chopped it roughly.

30g spinach leaves, remove the stalks

Red grapes 100g seedless

Cantaloupe melon, 100g peel it, cut into pieces

Instructions:

Blend all the ingredients into a juicer until it gets smooth.

Shakshuka Sirtfood Diet's – Breakfast

Total Calories: 299 - Serves: 1 - 40 minutes Preparation time

Ingredients

Onion, finely chopped 40 g; 1 Tsp Virgin olive oil; 1 clove of Garlic, fine-chopped ; 1 chilli, chopped finely; Celery, fine-chopped 30 g; 1 Tsp Cumin (ground); 1 Tsp of paprika; 1 Tsp Turmeric (ground); 30 g Kale, roughly chopped and stems removed; 400 g Tinned tomatoes (chopped); 2 Medium-sized eggs; 1 Chopped parsley

Instructions

Heat a deep fry pan over medium-low flame. Add oil in pan and fry for 1 to 2 minutes garlic, celery, onion, chili and spices. Attach tomatoes, and then allow the sauce to steam for 20 mins, occasionally stir it.

Add kale and cook another 5 minutes. Now if the sauce gets too thick, just add some water. Stir in parsley when the sauce has very fine, rich consistency.

Make 2 little sauce wells and pour all eggs into them. Lessen the flame to minimum and protect the oven with a cap or foil. Let the eggs for fry for 10 to 12 minutes, where the whites of egg must be firm whereas the yolks still liquidy. Cook another 3 to 4 mins if you desire firm yolks. Serve immediately.

Sirtfood Diet's Braised Puy Lentils

Total Calories: 310 - Serves: 1

Ingredients

8 Cherries, halved; Red onion, cut thinly (40 g); 2 Tsp Virgin olive oil; 40 g Carrots, peeled and sliced; 1 clove of Garlic, finely-chopped; 1 tsp of paprika; 40 g Celery, fine-sliced; 75 g puy Lentils; 1 Tsp thyme (fresh d or ry); 220 ml Livestock; 1 Tbsp Parsley, chopped; 50 g Kale, cut; Rocket 20 g

Method

Heat the oven 120°C/gas ½. Place the tomatoes in a tiny roasting pan and roast for 35 to 45 minutes.

Heat a casserole over low-medium-pressure. Apply 1 tablespoon of olive oil with garlic, red onion, carrot and celery and fry until softened for 1 to 2 minutes. Add thyme and paprika and cook it for another minute.

Wash the lentils in a sieve and attach them to the order. Bring to boil, reduce flame, and let it cook for about 20 minutes with a cover on the pan. Give the pan a swirl after 7 minutes, adding water if some amount fall too little.

Add kale and cook another 10 minutes. When baked, add in the parsley and roasted tomatoes. Serve with rocket with the remaining olive oil tablespoon.

Buckwheat Pasta Salad

Total Calories: 770 - Serves for 1

Ingredients

50 g buckwheat pasta (cooked packing instructions)

Pocket of basil leaves

8 Cherry tomatoes

Large rocket handful

1 Tbsp pure olive oil

1/2 Avocado

Ten olives

Instructions

Combine all the ingredients, except the pine nuts, gently and organise on a plate or in a bowl, then sprinkle the nuts over the top.

Sirt Muesli

Ingredients

10 g buckwheat puffs

20 g buckwheat flakes

15 g coconut flakes or desiccated coconut

15 g walnuts, diced

40 g Medjool dates, pitted and chopped

10 g cocoa nibs

100 g regular Greek yoghurt (or vegan substitute, such as soya or coconut yoghurt)

100 g strawberries, hulled and chopped

Instructions:

Mix all of the above mentioned ingredients together, and then add the yoghurt and strawberries before serving, if you make them in bulk.

Chargrilled Beef With Red Wine Jus, Garlic Kale, Onion Rings, And Herb Roasted Potatoes

----

Total Calories:: 707

Ingredients

5g parsley, chopped; 100g potatoes cut to 2cm cube; 1 tbsp virgin olive oil; red onion, (50g) cut into rings; 1 chopped garlic clove; 50g kale, sliced; 120–150g beef fillet steak/sirloin steak; beef stock (150ml); red wine (40ml); 1 tablespoon cornflour, mixed well in 1 tablespoon water; 1 tablespoon tomato purée

Method:

Oven heat to 220°C /gas 7.

Put the potatoes into boiling water in saucepan, bring them back to boil and prepare for 4 to 5 minutes, after this drain. Put 1 tbsp of oil into roasting tin, and roast for 35 to 45 minutes in the heated oven. Flip the potatoes after 10 mins to make sure cooking is evenly done. Take out of the oven when cooked, sprinkle the parsley on it and stir.

Fry the onions for 5–7 minutes over medium heat in 1 tbsp of oil, until it is soft and beautifully caramelized. Steam kale for about 2 to 3 minutes and drain it. Gently fry garlic in ½ teaspoon oil for just one minute, until it is soft not brown. Add kale and fry, until tender, for another 1 to 2 minutes. Hold on warm. Heat a frying pan which is ovenproof over high heat once it is smoking.

Cover the meat in ½ teaspoon of oil and fried over medium-high flame in a hot fry pan, depending on how you want your meat cooked. If you prefer your meat nice, it will be easier to fry the meat and move the pan to a 2200C / gas 7 set oven and complete the cooking as per the recommended times.

Take the meat out from the saucepan and set to rest. To take up any meat remains, put the wine in a hot pan. Bubble to probably lessen the wine, with an intense flavor, until syrupy.

Add the tomato and stock to the pan and take it to boil, and then to condense your sauce add the paste of corn flour, add a little of it at a time till the desired consistency has been achieved. Add any of the remained steak juices and eat with the baked potatoes, onion rings, red wine sauce and kale.

Greek Salad Skewers

Total Calories: 306 - Preparation time: 10 minutes -

Serves 1

Ingredients

8 cherry tomatoes; 2 wooden sticks; 8 black olives; Half red onion, half cut and divided into 8 chunks; 1 yellow pepper, sliced in squares; Feta (100g) cut in squares; Cucumber, 100g, cut in 4 pieces;

For dressing:

Virgin olive oil1 tbsp; Balsamic vinegar 1 tsp; Juice of half lemon; Half clove garlic, paste; Some basil leaves, chopped finely (or ½ tablespoon mixed dried herbs to switch oregano and basil); Some leaves oregano, chopped; Substantial flavor of salt and grounded black pepper

Instructions:

Connect each skewer in the order with salad ingredients: olive, basil, red onion, yellow pepper, feta, cucumber, lettuce, olive, red onion, yellow pepper, cucumber and feta.

Put the ingredients of dressing in a shallow bowl and fully blend together. Pour it on the skewers.

Chocolate Cupcakes With Iced Matcha

Total Calories: 234 - Preparation Time: 35 minutes

Simply amazing!

Ingredients

60g cocoa; 150g flour; 200g bran sugar; ½ tsp of salt; 120ml milk; ½ tsp of espresso coffee, decaf it if desired; ½ tablespoon vanilla extract; 120ml of boiling water; 1 egg; 50ml of vegetable oil

For icing:

50g of icing sugar; 50g of butter; matcha green tea powder 1 tbsp; 50g soft cream cheese; Half tsp of vanilla bean paste

Instructions:

Preheat the fan for oven to 180°C/160°C. Line a cake case with silicone cake cups.

In a large bowl, put the sugar, flour, cocoa, espresso powder and salt and thoroughly mix.

Add the dry ingredients with the vanilla extract, milk egg and vegetable oil, and use a blender to beat till it's blended. Pour it in the boiling hot water carefully and beat at low velocity until fully mixed. Using a fast pace beat to introduce air to a batter for another minute. A batter is considerably more solvent than a standard cake mix. Be confidence, it'll taste amazing!

In the cake instances, spoon batter equally. Each cake box is not more than 3/4 complete. Bake for 15 to 18 minutes in the oven, until the combination jumps back when squeezed. Remove it from the baking oven, and leave to cool until icing fully.

Cream icing sugar and butter together till pale and seamless, to end up making the icing. Attach the coffee and matcha powder, and then mix again. Add your sour cream, and then mix until smooth. Pip or sprinkle onto the cakes.

Sesame Chicken Salad

Total Calories: 304 - Serves 1 - Preparation time: 12 minutes

A delightful and rare salad.

Ingredients

1 cucumber, cut lengthways, seedless and sliced

1 tbsp sesame seeds

pak choi, 60g finely shredded

100g kale, chopped roughly

Half red onion, finely sliced

20g large handful parsley, finely chopped

Cooked chicken, 150g in shreds

For dressing:

1 tablespoon sesame oil

1 tablespoon extra virgin olive oil

2 tsp soya sauce

1 lime juice

1 tablespoon clear honey

Instructions:

Roast the sesame seeds for 2 minutes in the dry fry pan, until mildly brown and fragrant. Move to cool board.

Mix the sesame oil, olive oil, soya sauce, lime juice and honey together into a small bowl to prepare dressing.

Put the kale, cucumber, pak choi, parsley and red onion in a big bowl and mix gently. Pour over the sauce, once again combine.

Divide the salad with the grilled chicken between two bowls, on rim. Shortly before eating, sprinkling on the sesame seeds.

Aromatic Chicken Breast With Salsa, Kale And Red Onion

Ingredients

2 tablespoon of ground turmeric

120g chicken boneless breast

¼ lemon Juice

50g kale, chopped

1 tbsp virgin olive oil

Red onion (20g) sliced

50g buckwheat

1 tsp freshly chopped ginger

Instructions

Cut the eye off the tomato, and slice it very fine, taking care and have as much of the water as possible to make the salsa. Now, combine with the capers, chilli, lime juice and parsley. You might bring it all in a mixer however the end product is a bit special.

Oven heat to 220°C /gas 7. Now marinate the breast piece of chicken with the lime juice, turmeric, and a small quantity of oil in 1 tablespoon. Switch off for 5 to 10 minutes.

Heat the oven - safe frying pan, then attach the marinated chicken then cook on each side for about one minute or more until light yellow, then move to the baking oven (placed on the baking dish if your saucepan is not ovenproof) for about 8 to 10 minutes or till it is cooked through. Take it out of the oven, wrap in foil and keep to rest before serving for 5 minutes.

In the meantime, steam the kale for 5 minutes in steamer. Fry the onions and ginger in some butter and then put the fried kale and again fry for some more minutes, until soft but not colored.

Roast the buckwheat with the left over turmeric tablespoon, as per packet directions. Serve with vegetables, salsa and chicken.

Smoked Salmon Omelette

Try this fast and simple Sirtfood delicious dish riches with taste and heavens.

Ready time: 5 to 10 minutes -

Serves: 1

Ingredients

Smoked salmon 100 g, and sliced

2 eggs

½ tsp Capers

1 tsp chopped Parsley,

10 g chopped Rocket

1 tsp virgin olive oil

Instructions

Break the eggs in a bowl and then stir well. Put the capers, salmon, parsley and rocket.

In the non-stick fry pan, fires up the olive oil until heated but not burning. Attach the egg material and transfer the mixture across the plate, use a spatula, till it gets leveled. Lower the flame, and let cook the omelet through. Slip right the spatula along the sides and roll the omelet up or split in half and eat.

Sirt Food Miso Marinated Cod With Sesame And Fried Greens

Ingredients - Serves for 1

1 tablespoon mirin

20g miso

1 tbsp virgin olive oil

Red onion, 20g cut

Skinless cod fillet; 200g

Celery (40g)

1 clove of garlic, chopped

Kale, 50g chopped roughly

1 tsp chopped garden-fresh ginger

1 bird's eye chilly, chopped

green beans 60g

1 tablespoon sesame seeds

parsley, 5g, chopped roughly

30g buckwheat

1 tsp tamari

1 tsp grounded turmeric

Instructions

Blend the miso and mirin together with one teaspoon of oil. Dust the cod all over, then set for 30 mins to marinate. Oven heat to 220°C/gas 7.

For 10 minutes bake cod.

In the meantime, bring the left over oil to a large fry pan. For few minutes, introduce the onion and fry, and then incorporate the garlic, celery, ginger chilli, green kale and beans. Simply throw and cook up till the kale is fried through and tender. To help the cooking process, you have to put a small amount of water into the pan.

Cook the oatmeal with turmeric for almost 3 minutes in accordance with the packet instructions.

Remove the stir-fry with the parsley, tamari and sesame seeds, and eat with the shrimp and greens.

Raspberry With Blackcurrant Jelly

----

*Total calories:*76

Preparing a jelly beforehand is a best method to make the fruit hence it's prepared to eat 1st thing every morning.

Serves 1 - Preparation time: 15 minutes with setting time

Ingredients

Raspberries- 100g; 2 leaves of gelatin; Blackcurrants, cleaned and stalks are removed- 100g; 2 tablespoon granulated sugar; Water-300ml

Instructions

Assemble the raspberries in 2 dishes / glasses / molds to eat. Place the leaves of a gelatine for softening in a bowl containing chilled water.

Put the blackcurrants with water (100ml) and the sugar in a small saucepan and make them boil. Simmer hard for about 5 minutes, now turn off the flame. Leave for 2 mins.

Squeeze the leaves of gelatine to remove excess water and place them into the frying pan. Remove until completely dissolved, and then mix in the remaining water. Remove the liquid in the set dishes and set aside to cool. The jellies will be prepared overnight or in around 3 to 4 hours.

Apple Pancakes with Blackcurrant Compote

Total Calories: 337 - Preparation time: 20 minutes

Those are decadent yet healthy pancakes. A good lazy morning snack

Ingredients

Plain flour-125g

75g porridge oatmeal

1 tablespoon baking powder

A pinch of salt

2 tbsp bran sugar

2 apples, cored, peeled, and chopped into small chunks

2 tablespoon light olive oil

Egg whites (2)

300ml semi-skimmed milk

Ingredients you need for compote:

2 tablespoon caster sugar

120g blackcurrants, rinsed and stalks are removed

3 tablespoon water

Instructions

Get the compote, first. Put the water, sugar, and blackcurrants in a saucepan. Bring to a cooker and simmer for 10 to 15 minutes of time.

In a wide pot, put the oats, baking powder, flour, salt and bran sugar, then combine well. Mix in apple and whisk a bit at the time in the milk unless you make a seamless blend. Whisk the whites of egg to tight peaks, and fold it into the batter of the pancake. Bring the batter over to a tub.

Heat ½ tablespoon of oil over medium-high heat in the non-stick fry pan and add in around one fourth of batter. Cook until golden brown, on both the sides. Cut for four pancakes and redo to produce.

The blackcurrant compote pancakes fluffed away.

Sirt Fruit Salad

Total Calories: 172 - Serves for 1 - preparation time: 10 minutes

This sirt fruit salad is rich with one of the finest fruit SIRTs.

Ingredients

Honey 1 tsp

Half cup freshly prepared green tea

1 orange, split

10 red seedless grapes

1 apple, peeled and chopped roughly

10 blueberries

Instructions

Stir in ½ a mug of green tea with the honey. Once dissolved add half of the orange juice. Turn on to cool off. Chop other half of an orange and put the sliced grapes, apple, and blueberries together in a bowl. Pour over the leave and chilled tea to steep before serving for some minutes.

Sirtfood Bites

Ingredients

Dark chocolate-30g (85% cocoa solids) in pieces; or some cocoa

120g walnuts

Medjool dates 250g

1 tsp extra virgin olive oil

1 tsp turmeric ground

1 tsp cocoa powder

1 to 2 tsp water

Scraped seeds of 1 vanilla pod/1 tablespoon of vanilla extract

Instructions

Put the chocolate and walnuts in a blender and blend them until the powder is fine.

Remove all the remaining ingredients except water and combine until the blend forms a disc. Depending on the consistency of the paste, you do or do not need to apply the water-you don't like it to be so wet.

Make the material into the bite-sized balls using your hands, and refrigerate for almost 1 hour in a sealed container before you eat them.

In some extra cocoa or dried coconut you may round few of the balls to attain a better finish, as you just want.

Then keep it in your refrigerator for up to a week.

Tuscan Bean Stew

Ingredients

1 tsp extra virgin olive oil

Red onion, 50g chopped finely

Carrot, 30g, peeled and chopped finely

Celery, 30g trimmed and chopped finely

1 clove of garlic, chopped finely

½ chilli bird's eye, chopped (optional)

200ml vegetable stock

1 tablespoon herbes de Provence

400g Italian tomatoes, chopped

1 tablespoon tomato purée

kale, 50g roughly chopped

200g tin mixed beans

1 tbsp parsley chopped roughly

40g buckwheat

Instructions

Put the oil over low to medium heat in a small saucepan and fry the celery, carrot, garlic, chili, onion, and herbs gently while waiting for the onion to gets soft not brown in color.

Stir in tomatoes, stock and purée tomatoes and bring it to boil. Attach beans and require cooking for about 30 minutes.

Put some kale and then cook for the other 5 to 10 minutes, now add the chopped parsley, until tender.

In the meantime, cook buckwheat as directed by the packet, drain and serve with stew.

Salmon Sirt Super Salad

Ingredients - Serve: 1

Smoked salmon cuts, 100g (you may use lentils, tin tuna or grilled chicken breast too)

Chicory leaves (50g)

50g rocket

80g avocado, stoned peeled, and sliced

Celery 40g

Red onion 20g

15g walnuts, finely chopped

1 Medjool date, chopped and pitted

1 tablespoon capers

1 tablespoon extra-virgin olive oil

10g parsley, finely chopped

¼ lemon Juice

10g celery leaves or lovage, chopped finely

Instructions

Arrange the leaves of the salad in a big plate. Combine all the left over ingredients and top over with the leaves.

Kale And Red Onion Dhal With Buckwheat

Preparation time: 5 minutes - Cook time: 25 minutes

This Kale and Red Onion Dhal with Buckwheat is tasty and very healthy, simple and easy to create and naturally dairy-free, gluten-free, vegan and vegetarian.

Ingredients

1 tablespoon olive oil

3 garlic cloves, crushed or grated

1 small sliced red onion,

2 cm ginger, grated

2 teaspoons turmeric

1 chilli bird eye, seedless and chopped finely (extra if you love spicy things!)

2 teaspoons garam masala

160g red lentils

400ml coconut milk

200ml water

Buckwheat (or brown rice) 160g

100g kale (or spinach can be a good alternative)

Instructions

Place the olive oil in a dark, wide saucepan and add a sliced onion. Cook at low flame, with the lid on until softened for 5 minutes.

Add the ginger, garlic, and chilli, then cook for another 1 minute.

Add the garam masala, turmeric, and a sprinkle of water and cook for 1 minute more.

Add the coconut milk, red lentils, and 200ml of water (just by filling the coconut milk with water and tipping it in the saucepan in half).

Thoroughly mix everything together and cook over a gentle heat for 20 minutes with the lid on. When the dhal starts sticking, stir occasionally and add a little more water.

Add the kale after 20 minutes, whisk properly and remove the lid, then cook for another 5 minutes (1-2 minutes instead if you use spinach!).

Place the buckwheat in a medium saucepan about 15 minutes before the curry is ready, and add plenty boiling water. Bring water back to the boil and cook for 10 more minutes (or somewhat longer if you prefer softer buckwheat. Drain the buckwheat in a sieve and end up serving with the dhal.

Fragrant Asian Hotpot

Total Calories: 185 - Preparation time: 15 minutes

Ingredients

1 tsp tomato purée

10g Small handful parsley, finely chopped stalks

10g Small handful coriander, finely chopped stalks

Juice of ½ lemon

1 crushed star anise (or ¼ tsp ground anise)

500ml chicken stock, fresh or made with 1 cube

½ peeled carrot, and cut into sticks

50g beansprouts

100g raw tiger prawns

100g firm tofu, chopped

50g broccoli, cut into tiny florets

50g rice noodles, boiled according to packet directions

20g sushi ginger, finely chopped

50g boiled water chestnuts, drained

1 tbsp better-quality miso paste

Instructions

Place the tomato purée, star anise, parsley stalks, coriander stalks, lime juice and chicken stock in a large pan and bring to a simmer for almost 10 minutes.

Add the carrot, broccoli, prawns, tofu, noodles and water chestnuts and simmer gently until the prawns are cooked through. Remove from the heat and stir in the sushi ginger and miso paste.

Serve sprinkled with the parsley and coriander leaves.

Butternut Squash, Date And Tagine Lamb

Preperation time: 15 minutes - Cooking time: 1 hour and 15 minutes

Incredible Moroccan warming spices make this balanced tagine ideal for cold fall and winter times. For an additional safety blow, serve with oats!

Ingredients

2 tbsp virgin olive oil

2cm ginger, chopped

1 red onion, cut

3 cloves of garlic, crushed or grated

1 teaspoon red chilli flakes (according to your taste)

1 cinnamon stick

2 teaspoons of cumin seeds

2 teaspoons turmeric, grounded

½ teaspoon salt

800g lamb neck fillet, sliced to 2cm chunks

117

100g medjool dates, chopped and pitted

500g butternut squash, finely chopped to 1cm cubes

2 tbsp of coriander (and extra for garnishing)

400g chopped tomatoes and a half cup of water

400g tin chickpeas, boiled and drained

Couscous, Buckwheat, rice or flatbreads for serving

Instructions

Oven preheated to 140C. In a large oven-proof pan or a cast iron casserole plate, add around 2 teaspoons of olive oil. Attach the cut onion and cook onto a low flame until the onions are cooked but not dark, with the lid on for around 5 minutes. Attach the dried ginger and garlic, cumin, cinnamon, chilli and turmeric. Mix well, and cook the lid off for one more minute. If it becomes too dry add a drop of water.

After that, add in chunks of the lamb. Mix well to cover the meat in spices and onions, and then apply butter, chopped tomatoes and dates, plus around half a cup of water (100-200ml). Take tagine to boil, and then place the cover on and position for about 1 hour and 15 minutes in your preheated oven. Take out from the oven when the tagine is prepared, and mix it through chopped coriander. Present with couscous, basmati rice or flatbreads.

Note: If you really don't possess an oven - safe casserole dish or casserole of cast iron, only cook the tagine in any normal casserole before it needs to go into the oven then move the tagine to a standard casserole before putting it in an oven. Do an additional 5 minutes of cooking period to provide enough time to heat up the casserole.

Prawn Arrabbiata

Ready time: 35 to 40 minutes - Cook time: 20 to 30 minutes

Serves 1

Ingredients

125-150 g (Preferably king prawns) Raw prawns or cooked prawns

1 Tbsp Virgin extra olive oil

Buckwheat pasta: 65 g

For Arrabbiata Sauce:

40 g finely minced Red onion

30 g Celery, finely chopped

1 Clove of garlic, finely minced

1 Chilli bird 's head, finely sliced

1 Tsp Mixed herbs Dry

1 Tsp Virgin extra olive oil

2 Tbsp Blanc (optional)

400 g Chopped tinned tomatoes

1 Tbsp Parsley Cut

Instructions

Fry the garlic, onion, celery and chili over medium-low heat and herbs in the oil for 1–2 minutes. Turn up the heat to normal, then add wine and simmer 1 minute. Put the tomatoes and let the Arrabbiata sauce to cook for 20-30 minutes over medium-low flame until it gets a good rich thickness. If you are feeling the sauce gets too thick just add some water.

As the sauce is being cooked, let the water pan to boil, and cook pasta as directed by the packet. Drain, mix with olive oil when cooked to your taste, and hold in the pan till desired.

Attach the fresh prawns to the sauce and simmer for another 3 to 4 minutes before they have become pink and dense, then introduce the parsley and eat. If you use baked prawns, add the parsley, put the sauce to get boil and eat.

Mix the prepared pasta into the sauce and blend well yet gently and eat.

Baked Potatoes With Spicy Chickpea Stew

Preparation time: 10 minutes - Cooking time: 1 hour

The Spicy Chickpea Stew is absolutely tasty and provides a perfect topping of roasted potatoes, and as well as it also occurs to be organic, vegetarian, gluten and milk-free. So it has cocoa in it.

Ingredients

2 Red onions, shredded

2 tbsp. of olive oil

4-6 Baking onions, prickled everywhere

4 Cloves, rubbed or ground with garlic

1/2 -2 tbsp of chilli flakes (depends on how spicy stuff you like)

2 cm, dried ginger

2 tbsp of cumin seeds

Water-splash

2 Spoonfuls of turmeric

Tomatoes sliced with 2 x 400 g

2 x 400 g tins of chickpeas (or kidney beans, as you like) plus DON'T DRAIN chickpea juice!!

2 Teaspoons of unsweetened cocoa (or cacao) powder

2 Yellow peppers (or any colour!), diced in bits of bitesize

Top with salt and pepper (optional)

2 Teaspoons of parsley with extra garnish

Side salad (with option)

Instructions

Oven preheated to 200C, so you can create all the supplies you like. Place the baked potatoes in the oven when it is heated enough, and cook them for 1 hour or when they are cooked as you want them. Put the olive oil and diced red onion into a big broad saucepan until the potatoes are in the oven and cook softly, for 5 minutes with the lid on it, till the onions gets tender but not dark.

Remove the cap and add cumin, garlic, ginger and chili. Cook on low heat for another minute, then put the turmeric and a very little water and cook for another minute, and taking some care not letting the saucepan becomes too dry. Next apply cocoa powder (or cacao), chickpea (including chickpea water) and yellow pepper to the tomatoes. Take to boil and cook for 45 minutes at low heat up until the sauce is condensed and dried (but don't burn it!). Stew will be handled nearly at the very same interval as potatoes.

Finally, mix in 2 tbsp parsley, if you like, add some salt and pepper, and place the stew on the top of the roasted potatoes, maybe with basic side salad.

Choc Chip Granola

½ of your SIRT 5 a day

Total Calories: 244 - Preparation time: 30 minutes

Chocolate at breakfast! Be certain to serve with a cup of green tea to supply you with plenty of SIRTs. If you prefer the rice malt syrup can be replaced with maple syrup.

Ingredients

50g of pecans

200 g jumbo oats

3 Tbsp Olive oil

Chopped

Butter 20 g

2 Tbsp rice syrup with malt

1 Tbsp brown sugar

Strong standard 60 g (70 per cent)

Chips to deep chocolate

Instructions

Oven preheats to 160 ° C (140 ° C fan / Gas 3). Cover a large baking tray with a sheet of silicone or a parchment for baking.

In a wide tub, add the oats and pecans. Steam the olive oil, butter, brown sugar, and rice malt syrup gently in a medium non-stick pan before the butter has melted and the sugar and syrup dissolved. Do not let simmer. Pour the syrup over the oats and mix vigorously until completely coated with the oats.

Spread the granola over the baking tray and spread right into the corners. Leave water clumps with mixing, instead of just scattering. Bake for 20 minutes in the oven until golden brown is only tinged at the edges. Clear from the oven, and allow absolutely cooling on the plate.

While cold, smash with your fingertips any larger lumps on the plate, and then combine them in the chocolate chips. Place the granola in an airtight container or pot, or spill it. The granola is to last for at least 2 weeks.

GLOSSARY

[fonte https://en.wikipedia.org/]

Antioxidants: are compounds that inhibit oxidation. Oxidation is a chemical reaction that can produce free radicals, thereby leading to chain reactions that may damage the cells of organisms. Antioxidants such as thiols or ascorbic acid (vitamin C) terminate these chain reactions. To balance the oxidative stress, plants and animals maintain complex systems of overlapping antioxidants, such as glutathione and enzymes (e.g., catalase and superoxide dismutase), produced internally, or the dietary antioxidants vitamin C and vitamin   E.

Relation to diet - Although certain levels of antioxidant vitamins in the diet are required for good health, there is still considerable debate on whether antioxidant-rich foods or supplements have anti-disease activity. Moreover, if they are actually beneficial, it is unknown which antioxidants are health-promoting in the diet and in what amounts beyond typical dietary intake.

Autophagy: (or autophagocytosis) is the natural, regulated mechanism of the cell that removes unnecessary or disfunctional components. It allows the orderly degradation and recycling of cellular components.

Caloric restriction: Calorie restriction (caloric restriction or energy restriction) is a dietary regimen that reduces food intake without incurring malnutrition.

Circadian rhythm: A circadian rhythm is a natural, internal process that regulates the sleep-wake cycle and repeats roughly every 24 hours.It can refer to any biological process that displays an endogenous, entrainable oscillation of about 24 hours. These 24-hour rhythms are driven by a circadian clock, and they have been widely observed in plants, animals, fungi, and cyanobacteria.

Docosahexaenoic acid (DHA) is an omega-3 fatty acid that is a primary structural component of the human brain, cerebral cortex, skin, and retina.

Eicosapentaenoic acid (EPA; also icosapentaenoic acid) is an omega-3 fatty acid.

Gene: In biology, a gene is a sequence of nucleotides in DNA or RNA that encodes the synthesis of a gene product, either RNA or protein.

Hormesis is any process in a cell or organism that exhibits a biphasic response to exposure to increasing amounts of a substance or condition.[1] Within the hormetic zone, there is generally a favorable biological response to low exposures to toxins and other stressors.

Inflamm-aging: (also known as inflammaging or inflamm-ageing) is a chronic low-grade inflammation that develops with advanced age. It is believed to accelerate the process of biological aging and to worsen many age-related diseases.

Intermittent fasting: also known as intermittent energy restriction, is an umbrella term for various meal timing schedules that cycle between voluntary fasting (or reduced calories intake) and non-fasting over a given period. Three methods of intermittent fasting are alternate-day fasting, periodic fasting, and daily time-restricted feeding. Intermittent fasting may be similar to a calorie-restriction diet. Although being studied in the 21st century as a practice to possibly reduce the risk of diet-related diseases, intermittent fasting is also regarded as a fad.

Leucine: (symbol Leu or L) is an essential amino acid that is used in the biosynthesis of proteins. Leucine is an α-amino acid, meaning it contains an α-amino group, an α-carboxylic acid group, and a side chain isobutyl group, making it a non-polar aliphatic amino acid. It is essential in humans, meaning the body cannot synthesize it: it must be obtained from the diet. Human dietary sources are foods that contain protein, such as meats, dairy products, soy products, and beans and other leMaster Regulator: In genetics, is a gene at the top of a gene regulation hierarchy, particularly in regulatory pathways related to cell fate and differentiation.

Metabolism: is the set of life-sustaining chemical reactions in organisms. The three main purposes of metabolism are: the conversion of food to energy to run cellular processes; the conversion of food/fuel to building blocks for proteins, lipids, nucleic acids, and some carbohydrates; and the elimination of nitrogenous wastes. These enzyme-catalyzed reactions allow organisms to grow and reproduce, maintain their structures, and respond to their environments. (The word metabolism can also refer to the sum of all chemical reactions that occur in living organisms, including digestion and the transport of substances into and between different cells, in which case the above described set of reactions within the cells is called intermediary metabolism or intermediate metabolism).

Mitochondria: is a semi autonomous double-membrane-bound organelle found in most eukaryotic organisms. Tiny structures within a cell that break down nutrients and generate energy. They power the cell to carry out its functions. Muscle cells require a lot of energy, and so are particularly rich in mitochondria.gumes.

Polyphenols: (also known as polyhydroxyphenols) are a structural class of mainly natural, but also synthetic or semisynthetic, organic chemicals characterized by the presence of large multiples of phenol structural units. The number and characteristics of these phenol structures underlie the unique physical, chemical, and biological (metabolic, toxic, therapeutic, etc.) properties of particular members of the class. Examples include tannic acid and ellagitannin. Many foods in a healthy diet contain high levels of naturally occurring phenols in fruits, vegetables, cereals, tea and coffee. Fruits like grapes, apple, pear, cherries and berries contain up to 200–300 mg polyphenols per 100 grams fresh weight. The products manufactured from these fruits also contain polyphenols in significant amounts. Typically a glass of red wine or a cup of tea or coffee contains about 100 mg polyphenols.

Sirtuin 1: , also known as NAD-dependent deacetylase sirtuin-1, is a protein that in humans is encoded by the SIRT1 gene. SIRT1 stands for sirtuin (silent mating type information regulation 2 homolog) 1 (S. cerevisiae), referring to the fact that its sirtuin homolog (biological equivalent across species) in yeast (S. cerevisiae) is Sir2. SIRT1 is an enzyme that deacetylates proteins that contribute to cellular regulation (reaction to stressors, longevity).

Sirtuins: are a class of proteins that possess either mono-ADP-ribosyltransferase, or deacylase activity, including deacetylase, desuccinylase, demalonylase, demyristoylase and depalmitoylase activity.The name Sir2 comes from the yeast gene 'silent mating-type information regulation 2', the gene responsible for cellular regulation in yeast. From in vitro studies, sirtuins are implicated in influencing cellular processes like aging, transcription, apoptosis, inflammation and stress resistance, as well as energy efficiency and alertness during low-calorie situations. As of 2018, there was no clinical evidence that sirtuins affect human aging.

Stem cell: In multicellular organisms, stem cells are undifferentiated or partially differentiated cells that can differentiate into various types of cells and divide indefinitely to produce more of the same stem cell. They are usually distinguished from progenitor cells, which cannot divide indefinitely, and precursor or blast cells, which are usually committed to differentiating into one cell type.

Western pattern diet (WPD): or standard American diet (SAD) is a modern dietary pattern that is generally characterized by high intakes of red meat, processed meat, pre-packaged foods, butter, candy and sweets, fried foods, high-fat dairy products, eggs, refined grains, potatoes, corn (and high-fructose corn syrup) and high-sugar drinks. The modern standard American diet was brought about by fundamental lifestyle changes following the Neolithic Revolution, and, later, the Industrial Revolution. By contrast, a healthy diet has higher proportions of unprocessed fruits, nuts, vegetables, and whole-grain foods.

Xenohormesis: is a hypothesis that posits that certain molecules such as plant polyphenols, which indicate stress in the plants, can have a longevity-conferring effect in consumers of plants (i.e. mammals) and studies that relationship. It was first used in the paper "Small molecules that regulate lifespan: evidence for xenohormesis" by David Sinclair and colleagues from the Harvard Medical School. If the plants an animal is eating are under stress, their increased polyphenol content may signal forthcoming famine conditions. It could be advantageous for the animal to begin to react—i.e. to hunker down to prepare for the lean times to come. The effects researchers have observed from resveratrol may be just such a response.